Contents

Follow the rules

When you travel by car, always do up the seat belt. This is such an important rule that you have to do it by **law**.

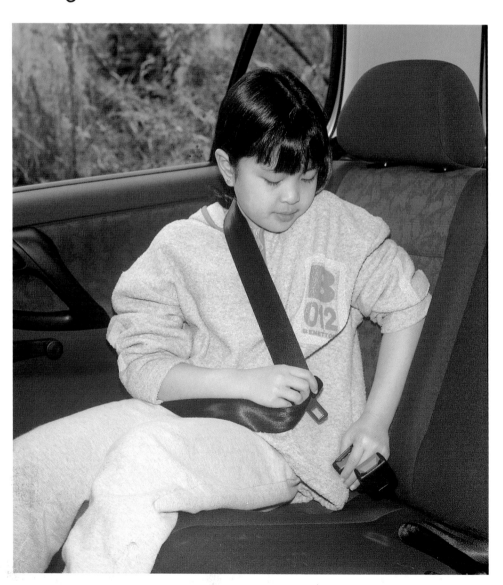

SAFE AND SOUND

Safety First

Angela Royston

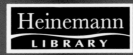

First published in Great Britain by
Heinemann Library,
Halley Court, Jordan Hill, Oxford OX2 8EJ,
a division of Reed Educational and Professional
Publishing Ltd.
Heinemann is a registered trademark of Reed
Educational & Professional Publishing Limited.

OXFORD MELBOURNE AUCKLAND
JOHANNESBURG BLANTYRE GABORONE
IBADAN PORTSMOUTH NH (USA) CHICAGO

Designed by Celia Floyd
Printed and bound in Hong Kong/China

03 02 01 00 99
10 9 8 7 6 5 4 3 2 1

ISBN 0 431 09144 7

British Library Cataloguing in Publication Data

Royston, Angela
   Safety first. – (Safe and sound)
   1. Safety education – Juvenile literature
   I. Title
   363.1

Acknowledgements

The Publishers would like to thank the following
for permission to reproduce photographs: Allsport:
S Bruty p10; Andrew Brilliant: p19; Bubbles: A
Compton p14, A Hampton p15, L Thurston p9, J
Woodcock p21; J Allan Cash Ltd: pp5, 17, 24, 25;
Trevor Clifford: pp4, 10, 18, 22, 23, 26, 28, 29;
Collections: J Greene p16; PowerStock: p20; Science
Photo Library: B Orchidee p7; Stockfile: p12, S Behr
p13; Tony Stone Images: R Daemmrich p27, D
Woodfall p6; Telegraph Colour Library: P von
Stroheim p8.

Cover photograph reproduced with permission of S
Bruty, Allsport.

Every effort has been made to contact copyright
holders of any material reproduced in this book.
Any omissions will be rectified in subsequent
printings if notice is given to the Publisher.

The Publishers would like to thank Julie Johnson,
PSHE consultant and trainer, for her comments in
the preparation of this book.

For more information about Heinemann Library
books, or to order, please telephone +44(0)1865
888066, or send a fax to +44(0)1865 314091. You
can visit our website at www.heinemann.co.uk.

Any words appearing in the text in bold, **like this**,
are explained in the Glossary.

Other rules and signs help to protect you at home, at school and outdoors. Follow the rules so you can play safely and have fun.

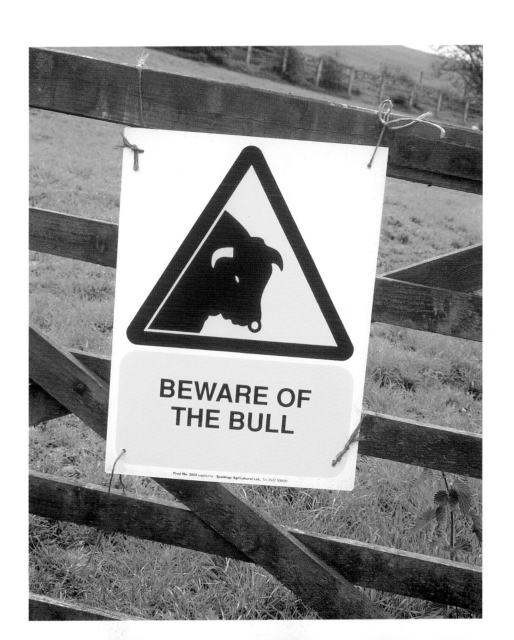

Poisons and medicines

This sign means '**Poison**'. Poisons can harm your body. Never touch or swallow them. Bathroom and kitchen cleaners often contain poisons.

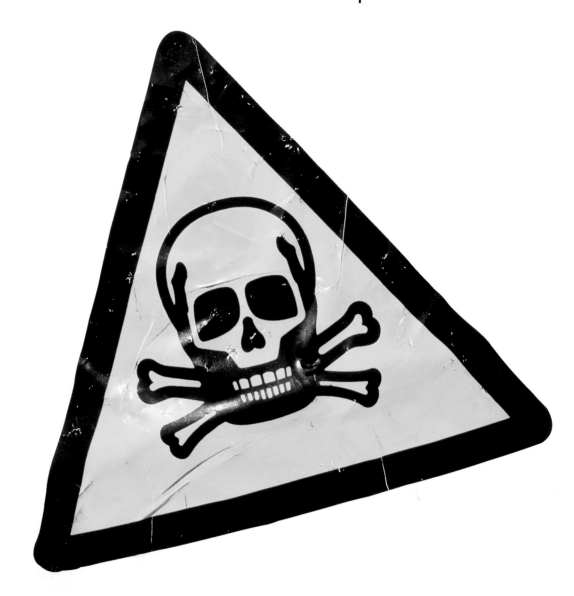

Medicines can make you better, but the wrong medicines can make you ill. It is very dangerous to swallow any medicines that are not meant for you.

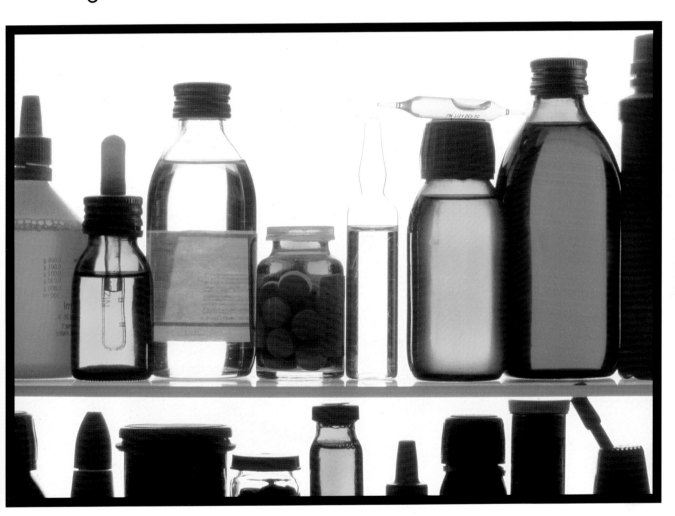

Crossing the road

Always walk on the footpaths, not on the road. When you have to cross the road, use a **zebra crossing,** or wait until the traffic lights show green for **pedestrians**.

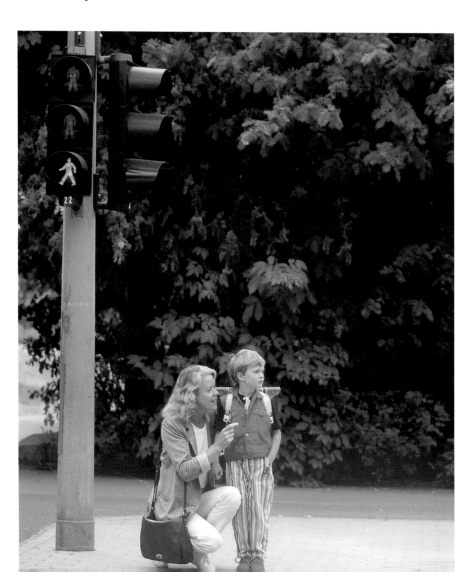

If the road does not have a special crossing, cross carefully. Wait until the road is clear. Listen out for **traffic** as you cross the road.

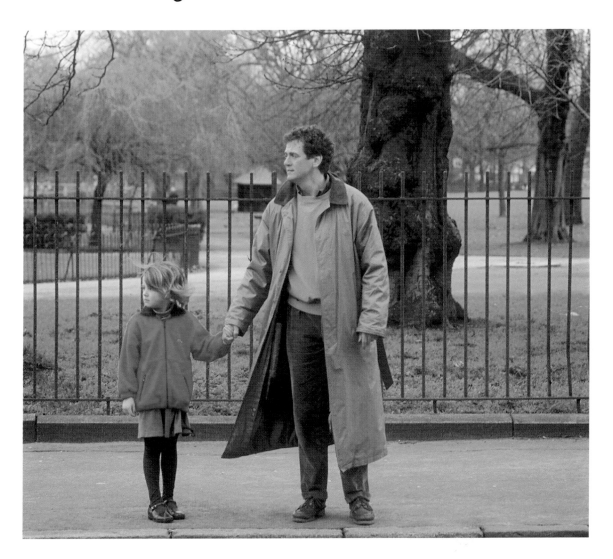

Dressed for action

These clothes are good for playing in. Jeans protect your skin and strong shoes protect your feet. Avoid clothes with strings that tie at the neck – they may **choke** you.

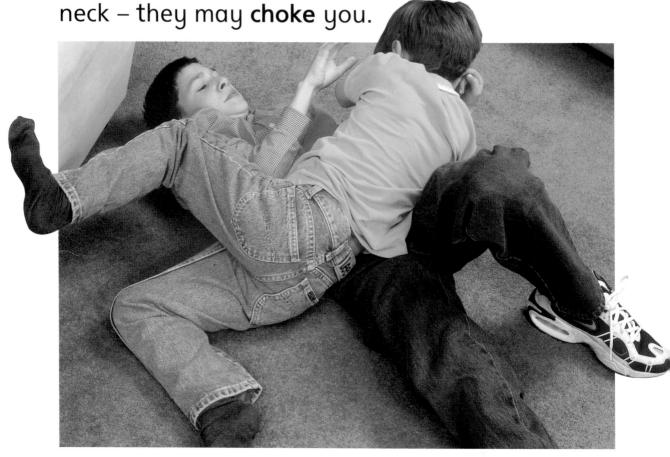

Do you like skating? Always wear a helmet and pads on your knees, elbows and wrists. That way you won't hurt yourself so much if you fall.

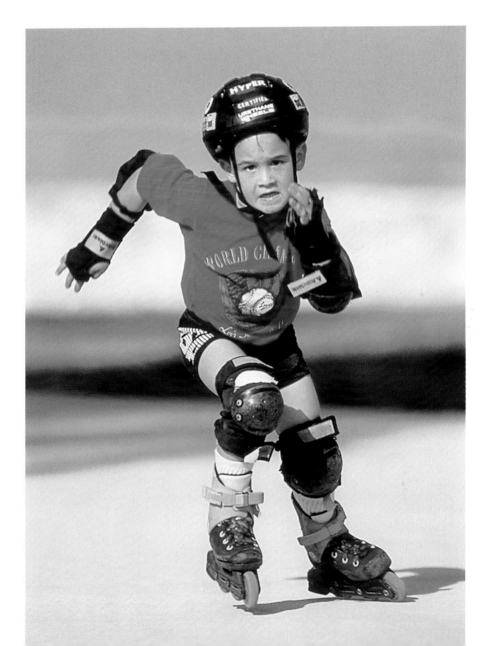

Safe cycling

Make sure you wear safe clothes when you ride your bike. Trousers or shorts are best because they won't catch in the wheels.

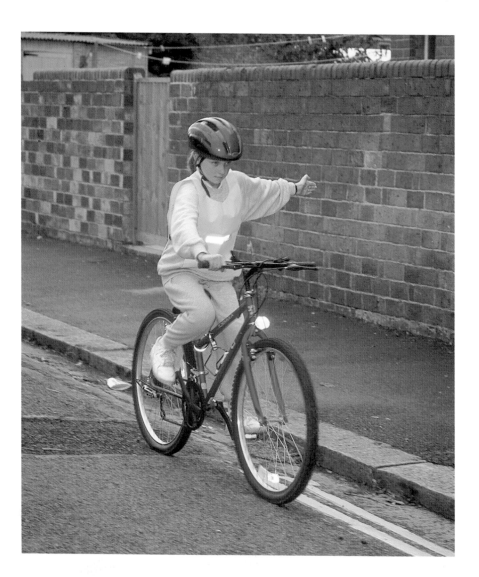

Always remember to wear a cycle helmet. This is the right way to put it on. The helmet should fit tightly on top of your head, not tipped to the front or back of your head.

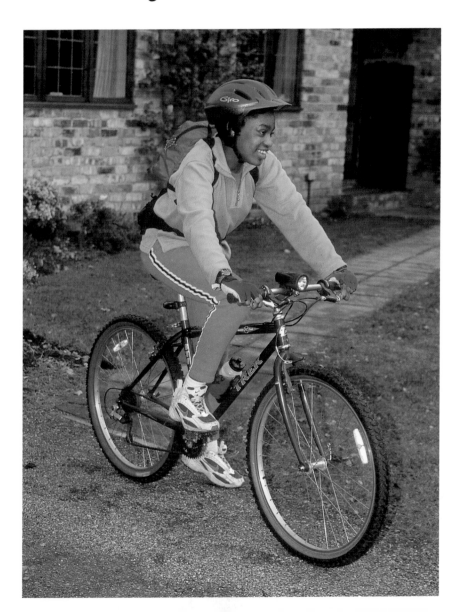

Covering up

Sunshine can damage your eyes and skin.
Wear sunglasses and rub in **sun cream** to
protect your skin.

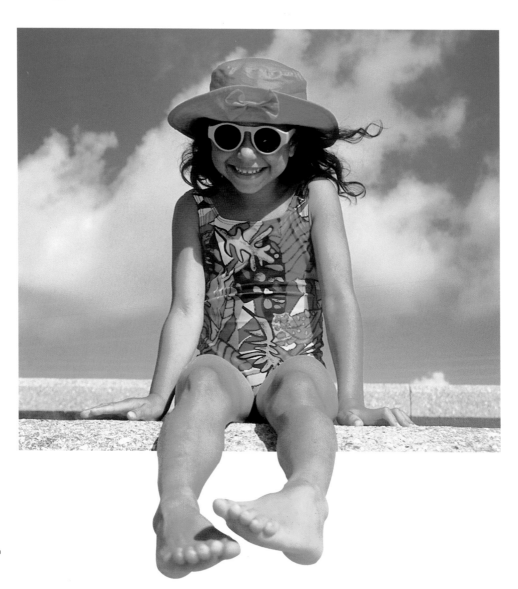

The sun is hottest for two or three hours before and after lunch. Stay in the shade then. Wear a T-shirt and sunhat to protect your skin and eyes.

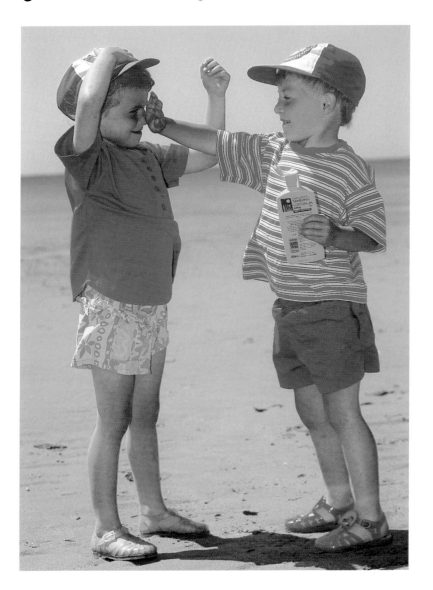

Safe swimming

Armbands keep you safe when you learn to swim. You should read and follow the rules of the swimming pool too.

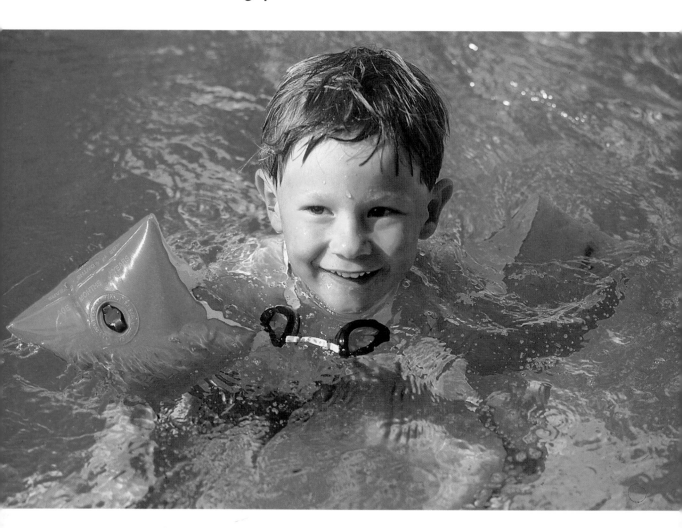

Some beaches have a **lifeguard** who watches out to make sure everyone is safe. Flags will often show which parts of the beach are safest for swimming. Even so, never swim out of your depth on your own.

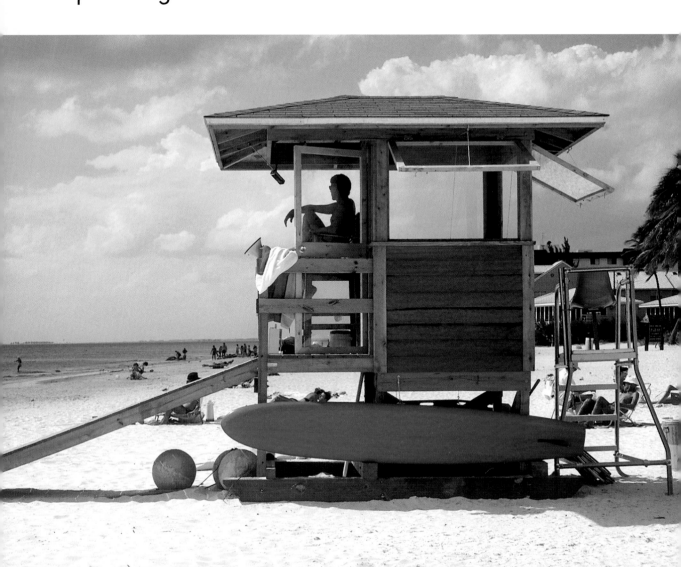

Water

If something falls in the water, stay on the side and use a stick to get it out. The water may be deep! Be careful of thin ice too.

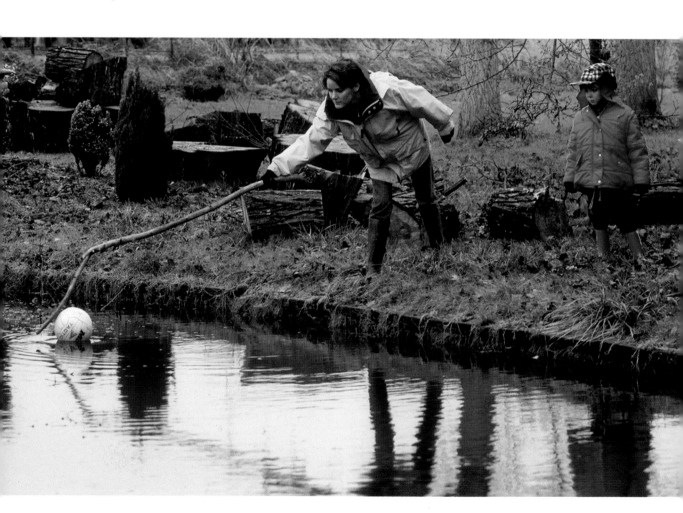

Wear a **life-jacket** if you go in a small boat or canoe, even if you can swim. The life-jacket will keep you **afloat** if you fall in the water.

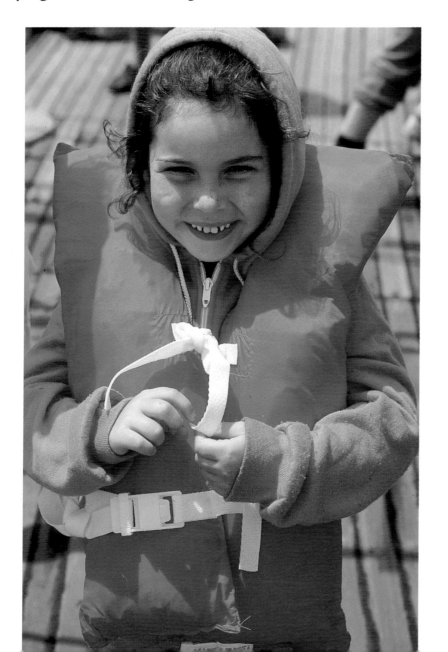

Fire alarm

It's easy to blow out the candles on a birthday cake, but matches can start fires that cannot be blown out. Never play with matches.

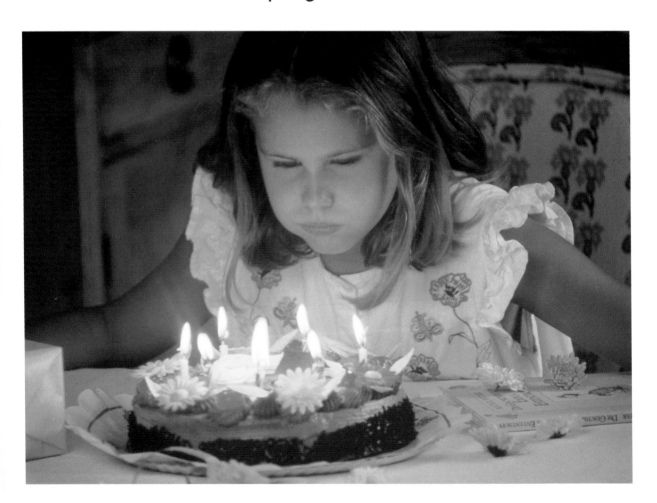

Many families have a barbecue when the weather is hot. Watch the food cooking, but keep well away from the hot, burning coals.

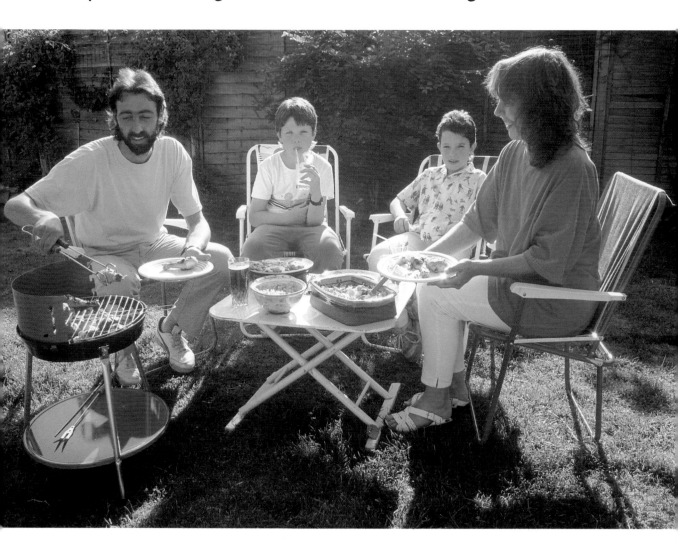

Electric shocks

Take toast out of a toaster with your fingers, not a knife. Never poke anything into electrical machines or plugs. **Electricity** can give you a dangerous **electric shock**.

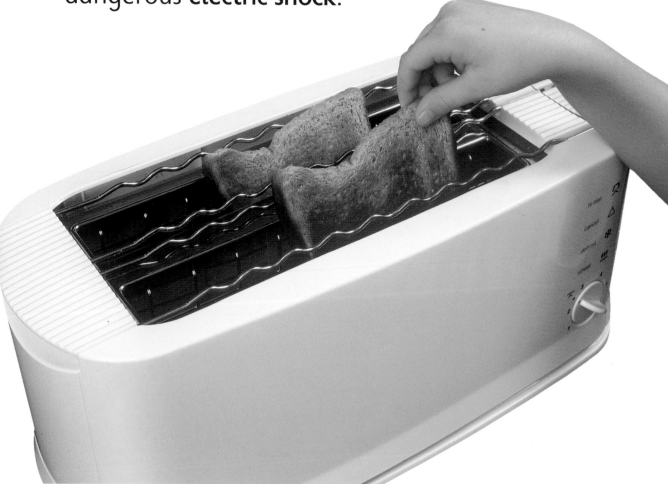

Be careful – electric irons, kettles and cookers can get very hot. They stay hot after they have been switched off, so keep away until they have cooled down.

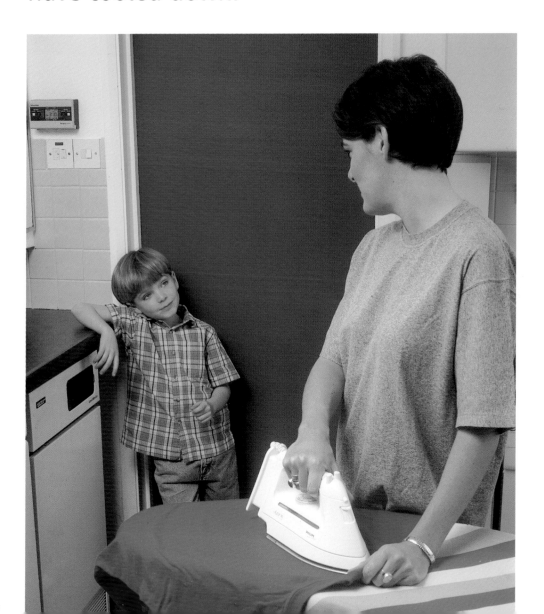

Play safe

A playground is one of the safest places to play. Other places, such as this building site, are dangerous for children.

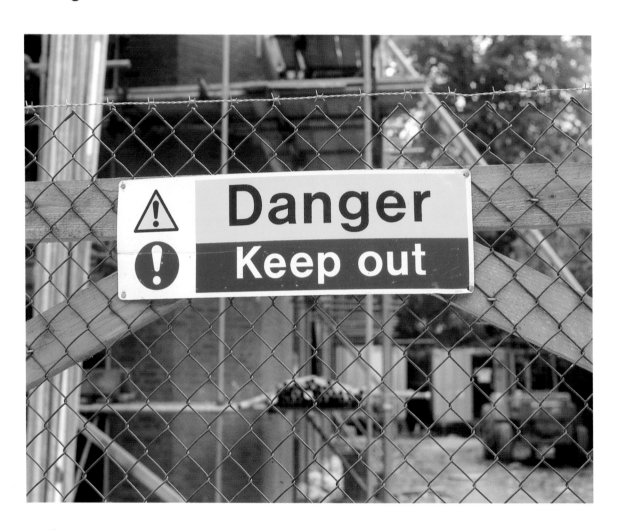

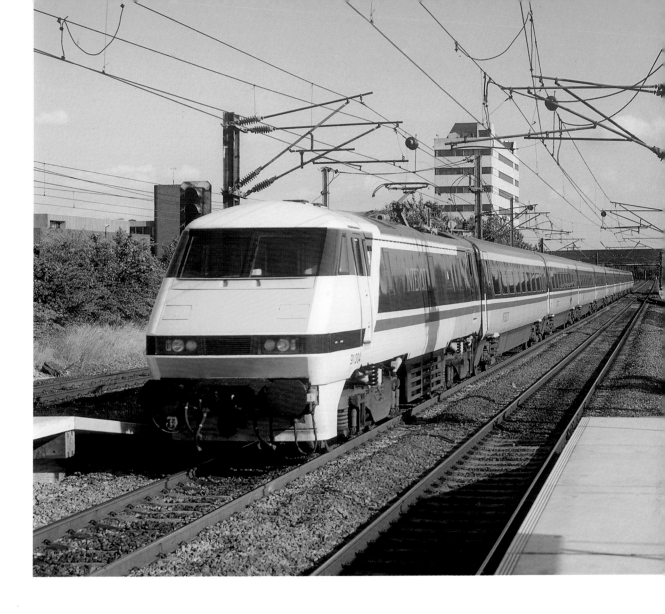

Keep away from railway lines. Trains travel very
fast and they cannot stop quickly. There may also
be dangerous electric **cables** by railway lines.

Keep together

Do not wander off on your own. If you get lost in a shop, tell a shop assistant. He or she will use a loudspeaker to call the adult you are with.

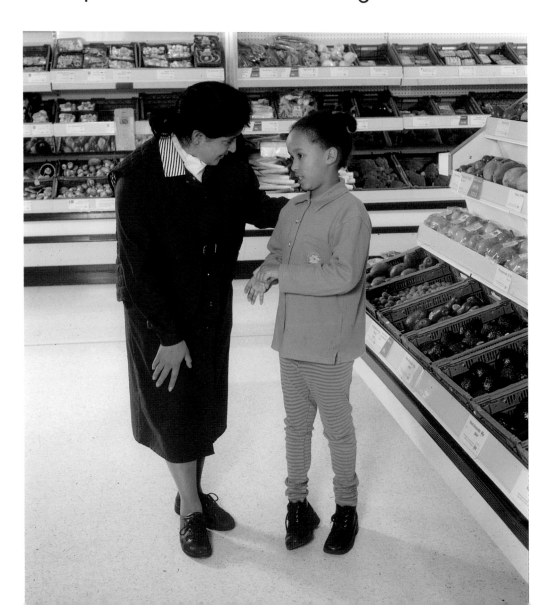

Some people are dangerous. If someone you don't know asks you to go with them, say no. Tell an adult and shout very loudly if you need help.

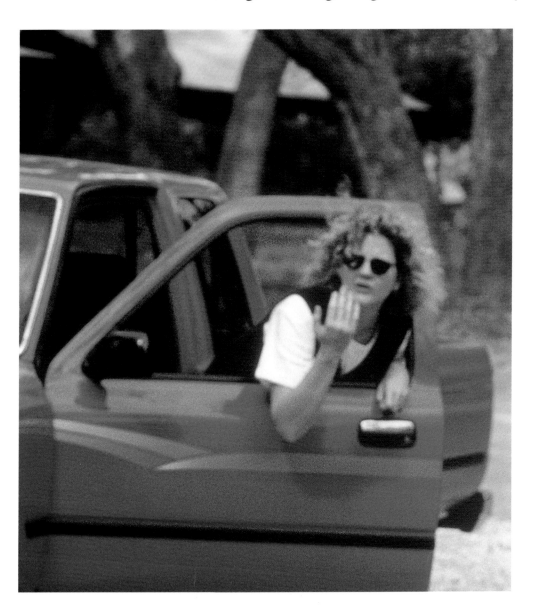

Getting help

The police, ambulance service and fire-fighters are always ready to help in an emergency. To call them, dial 999 and tell them where you are.

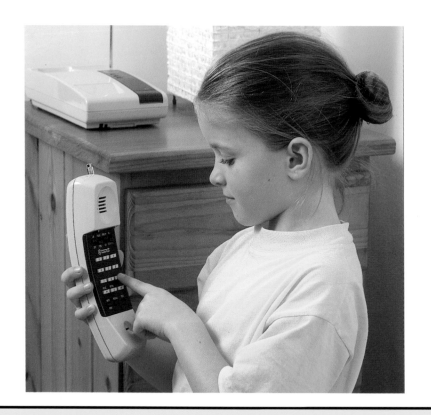

The emergency number is different in each country. In Australia it is 000. In the United States it is 911.

Don't let a grown-up or another child hurt you or make you do things you think are wrong. Tell an adult you trust, such as a parent or teacher.

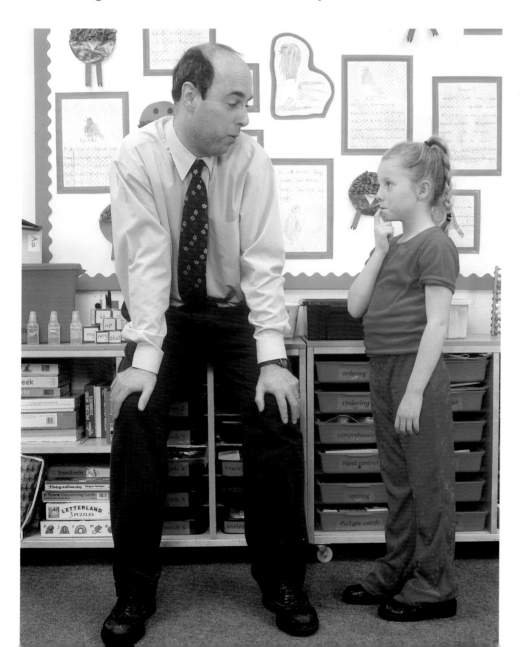

Glossary

afloat   on the surface of something, such as water

cable   thick wire

choke   not be able to breathe

electricity   some machines use electricity to make them work

electric shock   kind of injury caused by electricity

law   rules which everyone in the country must follow

lifeguard   person at a beach or swimming pool who watches out for people who might need help

life-jacket   special vest to keep you afloat, made of cork or other light material that cannot sink

medicine   things that ill people take to help them get better

pedestrian   someone who is walking

poison   substance which makes you ill or can kill you, if you swallow it or breathe it in

sun cream   cream that helps to stop skin burning in the sun

traffic   cars and lorries travelling along the road

zebra crossing   part of the road where it is safer to cross, shown by black and white stripes

Index